Wafa Dahmani
Nour Elleuch
Hanene Jaziri

Portfolio for medical interns

Wafa Dahmani
Nour Elleuch
Hanene Jaziri

Portfolio for medical interns

Designing a guide for gastroenterology department interns

ScienciaScripts

Cover image: www.ingimage.com

This book is a translation from the original published under ISBN 978-620-6-72726-2.

Publisher:
Sciencia Scripts
is a trademark of
Dodo Books Indian Ocean Ltd. and OmniScriptum S.R.L publishing group

120 High Road, East Finchley, London, N2 9ED, United Kingdom
Str. Armeneasca 28/1, office 1, Chisinau MD-2012, Republic of Moldova, Europe
Printed at: see last page
ISBN: 978-620-8-31027-1

ACKNOWLEDGEMENTS

To my Master and President of the Jury Pr Mehdi KSIAA

You have honoured me deeply by agreeing to chair the jury for my memory.

To my Master and Judge Professor Amina AOUNALLAH

I am honoured by the privilege you have given me to judge this present work.

To my supervisor Pr Ag Nour ELLEUCH

You have done me the honour of supervising this work and I hope that I have been able to meet your expectations. height.

No words can express my deep gratitude to you.

Thank you very much

Dear Masters,

Your scientific, educational and human qualities will be a great asset to me.

example to follow in the practice of my profession.

Allow me to express to you, through this work, the expression of my great esteem and my most sincere thanks.

TABLE OF CONTENTS

INTRODUCTION

Major reforms have recently overhauled medical studies in Tunisia, introducing a competency-based, student-centred and patient-centred curriculum. To adapt effectively to these changes, it is crucial to empower learners in their learning process, encourage the progressive and structured development of their skills, and offer them opportunities for self-assessment. These concerns have led to the search for solutions such as the creation of portfolios. The portfolio, which serves as both a learning and an assessment tool, has recently emerged as a key reference in training programmes for healthcare professionals (1).The integration of this tool into the training curriculum for medical students, particularly during their internship, is particularly timely. The internship, a pivotal period in medical training, is characterised by a high degree of autonomy and direct immersion in the hospital environment. The portfolio provides a structured framework to support interns in this transition, encouraging critical reflection and evaluation of their practices(3). It allows them to document the progress of their learning, to objectify the necessary adjustments, and to continuously measure the achievement of their objectives (2). However, until now, there has been no specific portfolio for interns, which could create a relatively significant gap in their training. The absence of such a tool could, in fact, deprive them of a structured framework for evaluating and improving their practice. The introduction of this portfolio is not only a step towards pedagogical improvement, especially as the portfolio has been adopted by our Faculty of Medicine in Sousse as a means of learning and assessing undergraduate students, but also a necessity in order to guarantee high-quality training in line with the contemporary requirements of medicine and the needs of students. The aim of this work is therefore to draw up a portfolio guide for interns at the Faculty of Medicine in Sousse assigned to the hepato-gastroenterology (HGE) department in order to implement it in the clinical environment.

MATERIALS AND METHODS

1. NEEDS ANALYSIS :

In order to design a portfolio guide that meets the specific needs of interns in HGE, we have implemented a two-stage approach:

1.1. LITERATURE REVIEW :

We first undertook a literature review in order to draw on empirical evidence and documented experience to design a portfolio that meets the specific needs of interns assigned to HGE.To do this, we carried out a literature search on the following subjects: medical education, portfolios, and the specific HGE skills required of a medical intern. We used the following databases: PubMed, MedLine, and Google Scholar, using the following keywords: Assessment, grading, Student performance, portfolio, Curriculum, Documentation, Competencebasededucation, Evaluation, Education, Medical Graduate, Internship, Gastroenterology, Competency.

1.2. ASSESSMENT OF THE CURRENT SITUATION :

To assess the state of training of interns assigned to the HGE department, we conducted an in-depth literature review.

Literature review :

➢ **Infrastructure and resources:** We examined the infrastructure and resources available in the HGE department at Sahloul Hospital, in particular the working conditions for interns and access to the equipment needed for their training.

➢ **Organisation of placements:** We analysed how placements were organised and managed, paying particular attention to supervision, interactions with patients and the diversity of clinical cases.

➢ **Training curriculum:** We studied the official documents and training guides provided by the faculty to identify the skills targeted and the teaching methods recommended.

2. PORTFOLIO GUIDE :

To design the portfolio guide, we followed the steps below:

➢ **Definition of objectives:** We have identified the specific educational objectives for the HGE placement and the competences to be assessed using the portfolio, formulated in a clear, specific, measurable, achievable and time-defined way to facilitate their assessment.

➢ **Structuring the portfolio**: The portfolio is designed to meet the specific needs of interns and encourage their professional development. It includes:

- An introductory section: general presentation of the portfolio, its purpose and how it works.
- A section dedicated to documenting clinical activities: interns are invited to document the clinical cases they have attended, focusing on their roles and what they have learned.
- A space for personal reflection: This space allows interns to reflect on their practices, identify their strengths and weaknesses, and formulate objectives for improvement.
- An assessment section: This is where interns record their formative and summative assessments, as well as feedback from their tutors.
- A space to showcase cross-disciplinary skills: interns can use this space to showcase the skills they have acquired outside a strictly clinical context (teamwork, communication, etc.).

RESULTS

1. RESULTS OF THE LITERATURE REVIEW

1.1. IDENTIFICATION OF GOOD PRACTICES :

We have identified a number of effective practices for designing portfolios in medical education. The articles analysed highlighted several key elements, which are summarised in Table 1.

Table I: Main Good Practices in the Use of Portfolios for Medical Interns

Nom de l'Auteur(s)	Année	Pratique	Description
Jia Yin Lim et al(4)	2023	Réflexion Personnelle	Cet article montre que la réflexion personnelle aide à intégrer les connaissances acquises en pratique clinique et améliore la compréhension des concepts médicaux.
T.Haldane et al(5)	2014	Récits de Situations Cliniques Complexes	Les récits de situations cliniques permettent de documenter et d'analyser des cas complexes, améliorant ainsi la résolution de problèmes cliniques.
E. Johnson et al(6)	2019	Feedback Structuré	Le feedback structuré améliore les compétences cliniques et la performance des internes. Les portfolios intégrant des sections pour le feedback facilitent le suivi des progrès.
Oudkerk Pool et al(7)	2018	Évaluation Basée sur les compétences	Les critères d'évaluation clairs permettent une évaluation précise des compétences des internes et facilitent la rétroaction.
Alomar et al(8)	2022	Apprentissage Multimodale	L'utilisation de divers formats de documentation enrichit le processus d'apprentissage et offre une évaluation complète des compétences cliniques et académiques.
Lisa Bußenius et al(9)	2022	Auto-évaluation	L'auto-évaluation encourage les internes à réfléchir sur leurs propres compétences et à identifier leurs points forts et faibles, favorisant un apprentissage autonome.
Tsekhmister	2020	Intégration de Cas	L'intégration de cas cliniques réels dans

et al(10)		Cliniques Réels	les portfolios permet aux internes d'appliquer leurs connaissances à des situations concrètes et d'améliorer leur prise de décision clinique.
Shrivastava et al(11)	2024	Le Tutorat	Les tuteurs jouent un rôle clé dans la guidance des internes, en facilitant la réflexion sur leurs pratiques et en fournissant des retours constructifs sur les portfolios.
Tochel et al (12)	2014	Évaluation Continue	Une évaluation continue à travers le portfolio permet de suivre le progrès des internes sur une période prolongée, offrant ainsi des opportunités d'amélioration continue.
Celis-Aguilar et al(13)	2023	Adoption de Plateformes Numériques	L'utilisation de plateformes numériques pour la gestion des portfolios simplifie l'organisation des documents, la gestion des retours, et facilite l'intégration des outils d'évaluation en ligne.
Lim et al(14)	2021	Décomposition des Compétences en Micro-Unités	En décomposant les compétences en unités plus petites et spécifiques, cette méthode permet une évaluation plus détaillée et plus facile à gérer, facilitant l'identification des domaines nécessitant des améliorations.

1.2. KEY COMPETENCIES IN HGE :

The literature review identified key competencies in HGE, divided into general and specific competencies. Among the general skills, interns must be proficient in conducting detailed interviews and physical examinations, prescribing and interpreting complementary tests, and communicating effectively with patients and the healthcare team (15). They must also practise critical reflection and self-assessment to continually improve their skills. In terms of specific skills, interns should be able to perform essential technical procedures such as ascites punctures and insertion of nasogastric tubes, and be able to diagnose and treat common and urgent pathologies in the EHG (7,16-19).

2. OVERVIEW OF

2.1. COURSES AT L'INTERNE

In Tunisia, training in general medicine takes place over six years, including an internship in the sixth year. This year is divided into four three-month placements in specialist departments, the main ones being Medicine and medical specialities, Surgery and surgical specialities, Paediatrics and Obstetrics and Gynaecology. Interns are allocated to HGE departments according to a ranking established by the Faculty of Medicine. At the end of their internship, their skills are assessed by means of an Objective Structured Clinical Examination (OSCE), which incorporates the knowledge and skills acquired during their various placements.

2.2. PRESENTATION OF THE SERVICE

HGE's services are organised into three main functional areas:

- **Hospitalisation**: to receive and monitor patients.
- **Outpatient consultations**: for outpatient consultations.
- **Digestive Endoscopy**: for diagnostic and therapeutic procedures.

The department's main activities include

- **Daily staff**: meeting at 8.30 a.m. to discuss new patients and ongoing cases.
- **Daily visits**: assessment and monitoring of inpatients.
- **Big weekly visit**: in-depth review of cases with the whole team.
- **Daily outpatient consultations**: treating patients on an outpatient basis.

➢ **Daily endoscopic activity**: carrying out endoscopic procedures.

➢ **Weekly staff**: presentation of complex cases and theoretical lectures.

2.3. Intern activity in the HGE department :

Analysis of the actual activities of HGE interns revealed a certain gap between theoretical expectations and daily practice. Although interns are supposed to :

➢ **Taking an active part in clinical activities:** Observations show that effective participation varies from one resident to another and from one period to another. Some are more proactive in patient management, while others tend to take a back seat.

➢ **On-call** duty: On-call duty is an essential part of training. However, the low ratio of interns to patients, coupled with the sometimes inadequate organisation of on-call duties, can lead to an overload of work for interns, to the detriment of their learning and well-being.

➢ **Performing technical tasks:** Opportunities to perform technical tasks are sometimes limited by the availability of supervisors.

➢ **Developing interpersonal skills:** While communication with patients is valued, interns do not always receive sufficient support to improve their interpersonal skills.

➢ **Working as part of a team:** Interns are integrated into the care teams, but the nature of their collaboration may vary depending on the team.

2.4. Assessment and validation of the course :

At present, the validation of internships in HGE is based on a qualitative assessment based mainly on the intern's attendance and general behaviour.

3. BUILDING THE PORTFOLIO

The educational choices relating to the content and organisation of the portfolio are based on the results of the literature review, while responding to the needs identified in the review, particularly in terms of the workload of interns and the resources available.

3.1. Definition of Objectives :

The general objectives of the portfolio are :

- **Facilitating the acquisition and assessment of specific skills**: Ensuring ongoing, in-depth assessment of clinical and theoretical skills, with an emphasis on practices and skills specific to the EHG.
- **Document learning in a structured way**: Provide a means of recording and tracking clinical experiences and learning throughout the placement, ensuring comprehensive and integrated evaluation.
- **Encourage constructive interaction between teachers and interns**: Use the portfolio as a tool to facilitate regular discussions and constructive feedback between interns and their tutors, thereby supporting reflective learning.
- **Enable continuous, dynamic assessment**: Provide an overview of skills acquired and progress made, by assessing performance over time rather than at a given point in time.

3.2. Contents of the Portfolio

The portfolio includes the following sections:

3.2.1. Introduction :

➢ General Presentation: Description of the portfolio, its purpose, and how it is to be used. Include clear instructions on how to complete each section.

➢ Learning objectives: Statement of the learning objectives that the portfolio aims to achieve.

3.2.2. Documentation of Clinical Activities :

Interns' clinical activities are documented mainly through :

➢ **Récits de Situations Complexes Authentiques (RSCA) (Stories of Authentic Complex Situations)**: this involves writing

detailed analysis of complex clinical situations encountered during HGE placements, such as rare digestive diseases or emergency situations. RSCAs should include:

▪ **A narrative account**: Describing the context and details of the clinical situation encountered, emphasising the challenges specific to HGE.

▪ **An analysis of the issues**: discuss the difficulties encountered and the study objectives, in relation to the clinical and technical skills specific to the HGE.

▪ **Research and summary**: Integrate validated information relevant to the case, with a summary of the learning acquired and skills developed (1.1, 2.2.1).

➢ **Questioning Clinical Situation**: this is a documentation of a specific problem encountered in HGE, such as an ethical situation linked to the management of a patient or a clinical dilemma. This section aims to promote critical reflection on complex issues (1.2).

➢ **Technical actions**: Recording of technical actions performed, with a description of the context, the technique and the results obtained.

➢ **Observations and Interactions:** Notes on interactions with patients, care teams and particular aspects of consultations or visits.

3.2.2. Personal Reflection :

➢ **Diary**: A space for interns to record their thoughts on their clinical practices, their strengths and weaknesses, and their feelings about the situations they encounter.

➢ **Improvement Objectives:** Interns should formulate personal objectives based on their reflections and feedback. These objectives should be SMART (Specific, Measurable, Achievable, Realistic, Time-bound).

3.2.3. Resources and References :

➢ This section includes useful resources for professional development, practical guides, relevant articles, and theoretical references that can help interns in their learning.

3.3. RATINGS :

3.3.1. Type of assessment :

➢ **Formative assessments**: represented by the regular assessments carried out by the supervisors, with detailed comments on the skills observed and suggestions for improvement.

➢ **Summative assessments:** overall assessment carried out at the end of the course, with a summary of the skills acquired and recommendations for the next stages.

3.3.2. Drawing up evaluation criteria

➢ Clinical skills: Assessment of technical and clinical skills based on precise criteria, such as correct performance of technical procedures and management of clinical cases.

➢ Interpersonal skills: Assessment of communication and collaboration skills with patients and the healthcare team.

➢ Reflection and self-assessment: Analysis of the intern's ability to critically self-assess and identify areas for improvement.

3.3.3. Assessment procedures :

➢ Regular feedback: Supervisors provide regular, structured feedback on the various sections of the portfolio, focusing on areas for improvement and successes.

➢ Use of an assessment grid: A detailed assessment grid will be used to assess the content of the portfolio, in particular the RSCA and the competences covered.

➢ Reviews and adjustments : The assessment criteria must be regularly reviewed to ensure that they reflect the training objectives and expectations of the various departments.

3.4. Portfolio guide for interns assigned to the HGE department:

A mock-up of this proposed portfolio is attached (Appendix 2).

4. IMPLEMENTING THE PORTFOLIO IN CLINICAL SETTINGS

4.1. Tutoring :

Tutoring is essential to the success of the portfolio and to the progress of interns, enabling them to :

➢ **Establish a relationship of trust**: Create a supportive environment where the feel comfortable discussing their difficulties and successes (7).

➢ **Clarify training objectives**: Explain the objectives of tutoring and the portfolio at the start of the placement, emphasising the skills specific to HGE (2.3).

➢ **Facilitating reflection and analysis of RSCAs**: Helping interns to write high-quality RSCAs, by guiding them in analysing and reflecting on the complex clinical situations they encounter (8).

➢ **Assessing progress**: Provide regular feedback on the skills acquired and the progress made. the evolution of knowledge, based on the criteria defined for HGE (2.4).

4.2. Integration into the Curriculum :

➢ Alignment with the curriculum: The portfolio must be integrated coherently into the training curriculum, with time set aside for reviewing and assessing the portfolio.

➢ Training of supervisors: Supervisors must be trained in the use of the portfolio and in portfolio-based assessment to ensure that interns' skills are assessed consistently and fairly.

4.3. IMPLEMENTATION AND FOLLOW-UP

Pilot phase :

➢ Portfolio testing: pilot the portfolio with a group of interns to gather feedback on its usefulness and effectiveness.

➢ Adjustments : Adjust the portfolio based on feedback received during the pilot phase to better meet the needs of interns and supervisors.

Deployment :

➢ Initial training: Organise training sessions for interns and supervisors on the use of the portfolio, its purpose and how to use it effectively.

➢ Ongoing monitoring: Regular monitoring to evaluate the use of the portfolio, resolve any problems and implement continuous improvements.

DISCUSSION

The internship is a crucial transitional phase in medical studies. To improve the training of interns assigned to the HGE department, we have developed a portfolio, the main aim of which is to inform their learning scheme and serve as a roadmap throughout their placement. This portfolio was designed to meet the various needs identified in our study, based on recognised best practice and taking account of the specific features of the Tunisian context, in particular within the EHG department at Sahloul Hospital.We will discuss the usefulness of the portfolio, examine its advantages, identify the difficulties and limitations of its use, and conclude with a look ahead.

1. WHY THE PORTFOLIO ?

The portfolio is a revolutionary method of acquiring skills because of the aspects of learning it enables to be assessed that are not accessible with other methods. These include self-training, self-assessment and reflexivity. This is a genuine paradigm shift away from transmission-based pedagogy and towards competency-based learning (20). It has become one of the new teaching methods, and the implementation of the portfolio during the various stages of medical studies, in this case during the internship, seems necessary (5,21,22).

1.1. THE PORTFOLIO AS A LEARNING TOOL :

With the shift in paradigms and teaching trends towards a participatory approach that encourages students to be autonomous in their learning, the implementation of active and modern teaching methods seems imperative. A number of training centres are trying to design portfolios as a means of learning. The aim is to regularly record the various achievements that are significant for the learner. It enables learners to follow their progress and helps them to become aware of their learning, through a kind of ongoing reflection/reflexivity and a critical look at what they have learnt and achieved(11,14). The idea of drawing up a portfolio for interns assigned to HGE services stems mainly from the fact that, until now, there has been no means of objectively tracing their achievements and situating the skills they have attained. This portfolio could also be used for all internships in the medical discipline, by being built around the cognitive, procedural and cross-disciplinary skills that an intern should acquire throughout his or her internship.

1.2. THE PORTFOLIO AS AN ASSESSMENT TOOL :

Various studies have analysed the use of portfolios in the assessment of healthcare professionals, exploring the ways in which they have been used for formative and summative assessments respectively, and examining the conditions for their accuracy and validity (12). A systematic review of the fidelity of portfolios in medical training reported a fidelity rate of 63%(23). In the context of high-stakes decision-making (national competitions, for example), a fidelity threshold of around 80% is sought; increasing the number of trained assessors would enable this threshold to be reached. A number of measures have a positive impact on inter-assessor agreement, including training for assessors, the use of small groups of trained assessors, consultation between assessors before (and sometimes after) the assessment and the use of criteria grids with qualitative descriptors (headings) (24). It is also advisable not to use the portfolio as the sole assessment tool, but rather to triangulate portfolio data with other assessment methods (OSCE or other)(12). The use of portfolios as a means of summative assessment also leads to greater adherence to the system. Indeed, several authors report that if portfolios were not formally assessed, their use faded. It seems that when attendance at portfolio work is not required, participants do not devote as much time to it (25).Through this work, we propose the implementation of the portfolio as a means of evaluation in addition to the OSCEs carried out at the end of the internship course. This would make it possible to take account of the intern's personal reflective work during the course and to obtain an endorsement of the skills acquired and those still to be developed.

2. EXPECTED BENEFITS FROM THE USE OF PORTFOLIO :

The introduction of the portfolio into the medical training pathway offers considerable advantages for both students and teachers.

2.1. FOR INTERNS :

2.1.1. Developing independence learning

One of the major purposes of the portfolio is to promote autonomous learning, which is essential for interns during their training periods. This autonomy translates into their ability to critically evaluate their own learning, identify their strengths and weaknesses, and direct their own professional development. This encourages a proactive, self-directed approach to learning, rather than relying solely on external guidance(5,26,27).

- **Capacity for self-assessment**: The portfolio enables trainees to record their clinical experiences, the cases they have dealt with and the skills they have acquired. By regularly reflecting on these elements, trainees can identify their strengths and areas for improvement. For example, by documenting a complex case of severe acute hepatitis, interns can assess their patient management, identify areas for improvement and adjust their practice accordingly.

- **Self-direction**: The portfolio encourages interns to take charge of their learning by setting personal and professional objectives. For example, an intern can set a goal for improvement in performing a proctological examination, and track their progress through the portfolio. This skill is crucial to their professional development, as it enables them to continue to progress throughout their medical career, adapting to new requirements and developments in the field.

2.2.2.Acquiring reflexive skills

Reflexivity is another major benefit of using the portfolio. It enables interns to develop a critical and in-depth awareness of their own practice and their professional development.

The portfolio provides a space for ongoing reflection on clinical experiences and learning(28). By regularly reviewing their practice and experiences, students can identify areas for improvement and develop strategies to address them.

By using the portfolio to reflect on clinical cases, such as the management of a patient with decompensated cirrhosis, interns can analyse their diagnostic and therapeutic approach. This reflection allows them to refine their understanding of best practice and treatment protocols, and to strengthen their ability to apply theoretical knowledge to complex clinical situations.

2.2.3.Improving professional practices :

The portfolio facilitates the integration of feedback received during supervision sessions. For example, after a discussion with a mentor on a case of colorectal cancer, the intern can adjust his or her practices on the basis of the advice and observations recorded in the portfolio. This ability to incorporate constructive feedback contributes to the continuous improvement of clinical and professional skills.

2.2. For teachers :

Teachers also benefit from the use of the portfolio, with well-documented advantages:

➤ **Improved interaction with interns:** Portfolios enable more in-depth interaction between teachers and interns. Portfolios serve as a starting point for richer and more constructive discussions between interns and teachers. With documents written by interns, teachers can engage in dialogue based on concrete evidence, rather than general impressions(29).

➤ **Knowledge of interns' needs:** Teachers can better identify interns' strengths and weaknesses. The literature indicates that portfolios provide a useful overview of students' skills, enabling more targeted assessment (12).

➤ **Curriculum knowledge:** Teachers gain a better understanding of the curriculum and its shortcomings. Portfolios can reveal aspects of the curriculum that need improvement, providing a basis for continuous improvement.

3. IMPLEMENTING THE PORTFOLIO: WHAT ARE THE CHALLENGES ?

The implementation of the portfolio, while promising, is not without its challenges. These obstacles can influence the effectiveness of the portfolio and its acceptance by interns and trainers.

3.1. Workload and Time Management

One of the main challenges is the additional workload involved in managing the portfolio. Residents, often with busy schedules and heavy clinical responsibilities, may perceive portfolio maintenance as a time-consuming task(30). To alleviate this problem, it is essential to design the portfolio in such a way that it fits seamlessly into their daily routines without adding an excessive burden. Solutions such as integrating digital platforms for portfolio management can help to make the process of documentation and updating simpler and more efficient(13).

3.2. Cognitive Load and Written Reflection: The Limits of the Writing Requirement

Despite the recognition of the value of the portfolio, a significant proportion of students feel that the requirement for regular writing in the portfolio generates significant stress. Some feel that reflection and analysis can be developed without the need for written documentation, and consider this additional task to be a waste of time that could slow down the learning process (31).

3.3. Training and consistency for Tutors

The effectiveness of the portfolio depends largely on the quality of the feedback provided by the tutors. Adequate training for tutors is crucial to ensure fair and constructive assessment. Tutors must be trained not only in the use of the portfolio, but also in the assessment methods based on it. Disparities in the application of assessment criteria can lead to uneven assessments and variability in feedback, which can affect the overall quality of learning (25).

3.4. Acceptance and engagement of

Acceptance of the portfolio by interns is another challenge. If the benefits of the portfolio are not clearly demonstrated, or if the benefits are not immediately visible, interns may be reluctant to commit fully to the process. It is therefore important to make interns aware of the benefits of the portfolio and to train them in how to use it effectively. Orientation sessions and concrete examples of how the portfolio can improve their learning and assessment can help overcome this initial resistance.

3.5. STANDARDISATION OF PRACTICES :

Consistency in the use and assessment of portfolios is also a major issue. It is crucial to define clear and consistent standards for the use of the portfolio in order to ensure uniform assessment of interns' skills across different trainers. Regular review of assessment criteria and use practices can help to maintain this consistency (28).

4.FUTURE PROSPECTS :

To maximise the benefits of the portfolio, a number of future prospects can be envisaged (11,28,29,32,33):

4.1. TRAINING FOR MANAGERS

Successful implementation of the portfolio will require adequate training for supervisors to ensure effective use of the tool and fair and constructive evaluation of the interns. Supervisors will need to be trained to provide detailed feedback and to use the defined assessment criteria, which addresses one of the concerns identified in our study.

4.2. WORKLOAD MANAGEMENT FOR INTERNS

It is essential to ensure that using the portfolio does not become an additional burden for interns. Strategies must be put in place to integrate the portfolio seamlessly into the interns' daily routine, without overloading their already busy schedules:

- Encourage interns to integrate their reflections on the portfolio into their regular activities, such as clinical case discussions or performance appraisals, so that it becomes a natural part of their professional routine.
- Developing a user-friendly digital platform for managing portfolios can simplify the documentation and updating of information. Digital tools enable rapid updates and easy access to information, reducing the administrative burden.
- Implementing automatic reminders for deadlines and updates can help staff stay organised without having to remember all the important dates.
- Design a simplified portfolio model that reduces the amount of documentation required, while enabling progress and skills acquired to be tracked effectively.
- Provide predefined templates and examples of best practice to help interns complete their portfolios more efficiently and in less time.

4.3. Ongoing assessment and Revisions

The portfolio should be regularly reviewed and adjusted in the light of feedback from residents and supervisors. This approach will ensure that the portfolio remains relevant and effective in meeting the training and assessment needs of HGE interns.

4.4. Longitudinal evaluation of Impact

Longitudinal studies should be carried out to assess the impact of the portfolio on the development of residents' skills. These studies could provide valuable data on how the portfolio influences the progression of skills and the improvement of clinical practice. The results of these studies could guide future adjustments to the portfolio model to better meet the needs of learners.

CONCLUSION

The current training of medical interns suffers from a lack of systemic planning, and assessment is often limited to a terminal and punitive aspect. This highlights the need for a more integrated and continuous approach. In this context, we have proposed a portfolio guide intended for interns assigned to the HGE department as an innovative teaching tool. This guide explains in detail the benefits of the portfolio, its content, how it can be applied and how to optimise its effectiveness. A pilot phase will be set up to test the proposed model, with adjustments planned based on feedback from users, to ensure its effectiveness and successful integration into the training curriculum.Although designed specifically for the HGE department, this guide could be adapted to the entire internship curriculum. By customising the assessment criteria and content for each speciality, this initiative could harmonise teaching practices within the Sousse Faculty of Medicine, while promoting the acquisition of solid and lasting professional skills for future doctors.

REFERENCES

1. Naccache N, Samson L, Jouquan J. Le portfolio en éducation des sciences de la santé: un outil d'apprentissage, de développement professionnel et d'évaluation. Pédagogie Médicale. May 2006;7(2):110-27.

2. Amsellem-Ouazana D, Pee DV, Godin V. Use of portfolios as a learning and assessment tool in a surgical practical session of urology during undergraduate medical training. Medical Teacher. Jan 2006;28(4):356-9.

3. Buckley S, Coleman J, Davison I, S. Khan K, Zamora J, Malick S, et al. The educational effects of portfolios on student learning during the undergraduate curriculum: a systematic review from the Best Evidence Medical Education (BEME) collaboration. BEME Guide No. 11. Pédagogie Médicale. May 2012;13(2):115-45.

4. Lim JY, Ong SYK, Ng CYH, Chan KLE, Wu SYEA, So WZ, et al. A systematic scoping review of reflective writing in medical education. BMC Med Educ. 9 Jan 2023;23(1):12.

5. Haldane T. 'Portfolios' as a method of assessment in medical education. Gastroenterol Hepatol Bed Bench. 2014;7(2):89-93.

6. Johnson CE, Keating JL, Farlie MK, Kent F, Leech M, Molloy EK. Educators' behaviours during feedback in authentic clinical practice settings: an observational study and systematic analysis. BMC Med Educ. Dec 2019;19(1):129.

7. A. OP. Competency-based portfolio assessment: unraveling stakeholder perspectives and assessment practices [Internet]. maastricht university; 2020 [cited 27 Aug 2024]. Available from: https://cris.maastrichtuniversity.nl/en/publications/6e14e871-22a6-49e4- ae53-b108f3375ead

8. Alomar AZ. A structured multimodal teaching approach enhancing

musculoskeletal physical examination skills among undergraduate medical students. Med Educ Online. Dec 2022;27(1):2114134.

9. Bußenius L, Harendza S, Van Den Bussche H, Selch S. Final-year medical students' self-assessment of facets of competence for beginning residents. BMC Med Educ. 7 Feb 2022;22(1):82.

10. Tsekhmister Y. Effectiveness of case-based learning in medical and pharmacy education: A meta-analysis. ELECTRON J GEN MED. 1 Sep 2023;20(5):em515.

11. Shrivastava SR, Maulida AP. Streamlining Medical Journey: Leveraging Portfolios for Mentoring Medical Students. Journal of the Scientific Society. 2024;51(1):3-6.

12. Tochel C, Haig A, Hesketh A, Cadzow A, Beggs K, Colthart I, et al. The effectiveness of portfolios for assessment and training during the postgraduate curriculum. BEME Guide No. 12. medical pedagogy. may 2014;15(2):113-48.

13. Celis-Aguilar E, Ruiz-Xicoténcatl J. Conventional and electronic portfolios in medical residencies. Educación Médica. Sep 2018;19(5):309-15.

14. Lim AJS, Hong DZ, Pisupati A, Ong YT, Yeo JYH, Chong EJX, et al. Portfolio use in postgraduate medical education: a systematic scoping review. Postgraduate Medical Journal. 21 Jul 2023;99(1174):913-27.

15. Final+4687 (1).pdf.

16. Kadokawa Y, Katayama K, Takahashi K, Fukushima N, Tanaka S, Taniguchi Y, et al. The Effectiveness of a Liver Disease Education Class for Providing Information to Patients and Their Families. J Clin Med Res. 2017;9(3):207-12.

17. Tazinkeng N, Monteiro JFG, Thomson SR, David Y, Madkour A, Katsidzira L, et al. Gastroenterology training in Africa: an assessment of curriculum and perception. The Lancet Gastroenterology & Hepatology. March 2024;9(3):195-7.

18. Gastroenterology Curriculum. 2019;
19. gastroenterology-selective.pdf.
20. Huenges B, Woestmann B, Ruff-Dietrich S, Rusche H. Self-Assessment of competence during post-graduate training in general medicine: A preliminary study to develop a portfolio for further education. GMS Journal for Medical Education; 34(5):Doc68 [Internet]. 15 Nov 2017 [cited 29 Aug 2024]; Available from: http://www.egms.de/en/journals/zma/2017-34/zma001145.shtml
21. Challis M, Mathers NJ, Howe AC, Field NJ. Portfolio-based learning: continuing medical education for general practitioners - a mid-point evaluation. Medical Education. Jan 1997;31(1):22-6.
22. Long DM. Competency-based Residency Training: The Next Advance in Graduate Medical Education. Academic Medicine. Dec 2000;75(12):1178-83.
23. McCready T. Portfolios and the assessment of competence in nursing: A literature review. International Journal of Nursing Studies. Jan 2007;44(1):143-51.
24. Driessen E, Van Tartwijk J, Van Der Vleuten C, Wass V. Portfolios in medical education: why do they meet with mixed success? A systematic review: portfolios. Medical Education. 28 Nov 2007;41(12):1224-33.
25. Pearson DJ, Heywood P. Portfolio use in general practice vocational training: a survey of GP registrars. Med Educ. Jan 2004;38(1):87-95.
26. Tochel C, Haig A, Hesketh A, Cadzow A, Beggs K, Colthart I, et al. The effectiveness of portfolios for postgraduate assessment and education: BEME Guide No 12. Medical Teacher. Jan 2009;31(4):299-318.
27. Thomé G, Hovenberg H, Edgren G. Portfolio as a method for continuous assessment in an undergraduate health education programme. Medical Teacher. Jan 2006;28(6):e171-6.
28. Girardot D, Lambert C, Ratelle R. Conditions for implementing the electronic portfolio"Aristotle in a specialty training programme: a pilot study in

radio-oncology. Pédagogie Médicale. Nov 2010;11(4):213-24.

29. McEwen LA, Griffiths J, Schultz K. Developing and Successfully Implementing a Competency-Based Portfolio Assessment System in a Postgraduate Family Medicine Residency Program: Academic Medicine. nov 2015;90(11):1515-26.

30. Elango S, Jutti RC, Lee LK. Portfolio as a learning tool: students' perspective. Ann Acad Med Singap. Sept 2005;34(8):511-4.

31. Finlay, Maughan, Webster. A randomized controlled study of portfolio learning in undergraduate cancer education: Portfolio learning in cancer education. Medical Education. Apr 1998;32(2):172-6.

32. Pitts J, Coles C, Thomas P, Smith F. Enhancing reliability in portfolio assessment: discussions between assessors. Medical Teacher. Jan 2002;24(2):197-201.

33. Davis C, Curzio J. Avoiding the pitfalls of Action Learning. Nurse Education in Practice. Dec 2003;3(4):183-4.

APPENDICES

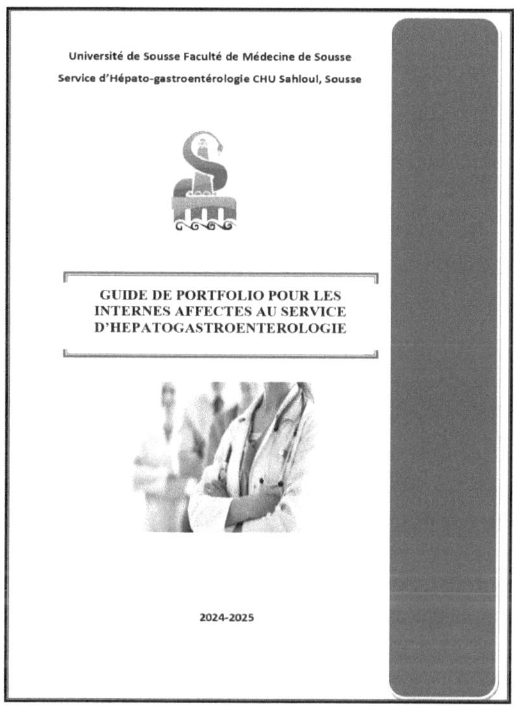

"This portfolio will be your travelling companion throughout your training period in Hepato-Gastro-Enterology. It will enable you to document your learning, reflect on your practices and build your professional identity. It's much more than just a collection of documents; it's a tool for empowerment, a space for dialogue with yourself and your supervisors.

WELCOME

"The team at the Hepatogastroenterology Department welcomes you. During this placement, you will become familiar with frequent medical situations of varying difficulty, take an active part in patient management and acquire essential technical skills. Your apprenticeship will be all the more effective if you demonstrate discipline, rigour, professional awareness and a sense of how to relate to patients and the care team. Your commitment and curiosity will be the keys to your success, and we are committed to supporting you throughout your apprenticeship.

INTERNSHIP IN THE HEPATO GASTROENTEROLOGY DEPARTMENT

Hepato-Gastroenterology is a vast and versatile speciality, encompassing the medical management of all diseases of the digestive tract and covering multiple organs (digestive tract from oesophagus to anus, liver and biliary tract, pancreas, peritoneum) through a multidisciplinary prism (inflammatory diseases, infectious diseases, nutritional management, oncology, management of chronic diseases, digestive motor disorders, etc.).). This is a medical-interventional speciality in which endoscopy plays a key role. "The Sahloul Hepato-Gastro-Enterology Department offers you a complete immersion in the world of gastroenterology. At the heart of our unit, which has 7 rooms and a dynamic endoscopy unit, you will be involved in patient care.Our organisation, with daily staff meetings and regular on-call duty, will enable you to develop your clinical skills gradually. Every DAY, you will be confronted with a variety of cases, enabling you to gain solid experience and develop your critical thinking skills.

Department activity

• **Staff organisation chart**: The daily medical staff meeting begins at 8.30am, marking the start of the working day. On-call cases are discussed at these meetings. You will be asked to present the files of patients admitted during the shift or those who have developed complications. On Tuesdays, a special meeting is organised to discuss problem cases, followed by a bibliography session or presentation of a clinical case by one of the residents.

• **Day activity**: After the morning staff meeting, each extern, intern and resident must go to their shift according to the established distribution. You will be responsible for your patients and for keeping their records. Each senior doctor makes a daily visit to his or her sector, and you will be expected to present the cases for which you are responsible. Attendance is compulsory and presentation of cases is required.

• **On-call duty**: As an intern, you will be required to work on-call in pairs with a resident, under the responsibility of a senior doctor. This experience will enable you to put your knowledge into practice and gain greater autonomy in managing emergency situations.

COMPETENCES TO AIM FOR

During this placement, you will develop and refine a range of skills that are essential for your future practice in medicine. These are the skills you will need to master:

1. **General powers** :

• Mastery of the Scientific Foundations: You will need to have an in-depth understanding of the scientific foundations relating to digestive pathologies, including the anatomy, physiology and biochemistry of the digestive system. Make sure you are familiar with pharmacology and microbiology concepts relevant to informed practice.

• Application of the Scientific Method: You will learn to formulate hypotheses, conduct bibliographical research and interpret data rigorously. These skills are crucial for evidence-based clinical decision-making.

• Professional communication: You will need to develop effective communication skills with patients, their families and members of the medical team. The ability to convey information clearly and empathetically is essential.

• Teamwork: Modern medicine is often a team affair. You'll be working with a variety of health professionals, and it's important to be able to work harmoniously as part of that team.

• Respect for ethical principles: Ethics and professional conduct are at the heart of medical practice. You must always respect ethical principles and demonstrate professionalism in your interactions with patients and colleagues.

2. **Specific HGE skills** :

- Medical history and physical examination: You'll need to excel at collecting and analysing data. medical history and in carrying out comprehensive clinical examinations, including the proctological examinations required to assess specific pathologies.
- Paraclinical exploration: Interpreting biological results, imaging tests and endoscopic procedures will be a key part of your training. Make sure you master these skills for an accurate diagnosis.
- Diagnosis: You will be trained to make accurate diagnoses, particularly in digestive emergencies. You will also need to know how to establish differential diagnoses in order to guide appropriate treatment.
- Therapeutics: You will learn to prescribe and manage treatments for various digestive pathologies. Understanding treatment options and the ability to tailor treatment to individual patient needs will be essential.
- Prevention: Prevention is an important part of medicine. You will be trained to identify risk factors, promote healthy lifestyle habits and carry out effective screening.
- Technical procedures: Mastery of technical procedures, such as ascites puncture and nasogastric tube placement, is an integral part of your skills. You will be required to practise and master these techniques under supervision.

We look forward to watching you progress and supporting your professional development throughout the course.

We wish you every success,

The Hepatogastroenterology Department Team

HOW TO CREATE A PORTFOLIO

The following document is a guide to help you create an effective portfolio that represents your placement experience. Here are the essential steps and elements for creating a portfolio that will enable you to track your progress and illustrate your achievements.

-What is a portfolio?

A portfolio is a documentation tool used to :

• Collect and organise a variety of data relating to your learning and achievements.

• Report on your work, highlighting your effo1ts, progress and achievements.

• Provide a critical analysis of your content, allowing you to step back and evaluate your work.

-Why use a portfolio?

A portfolio offers several avm1tages:

• Consolidation of learning: By bringing all your tools and documents together in one place, you can monitor your progress and identify any difficulties encountered.

• Personal expression: As well as an exam, a p01tfolio allows you to show off your creativity and personality.

• Reflection and self-assessment: By reflecting on the documents you choose to include, you develop a reflective process that helps you assess your skills and progress.

-How do you create a portfolio?

Here are the key stages in developing a p01tfolio:

Document selection : Choose the most significant learning h-spaces related to the development of your skills. These documents can include summaries, diagrams, tables, videos, etc.

2. Justification of documents : Each document included must be preceded by an explanation of its interest and relevance to your learning.

3. Critical reflection: After each document, write a personal reflection on what you have read. what you have learned and how this contributes to your professional development. Your portfolio should reflect your achievements and progress, while highlighting your personal qualities.

-How should your portfolio be structured?

The portfolio can be structured as follows, although you can customise this structure to suit your needs:

1. **Identification sheet**
2. **Learning activities**
3. **Skills to aim for**
4. **Library and personal research**
5. **Internship report**
6. **Open comments, outlook**

These different parts are detailed below.

• **Portfolio format**

Various formats exist (paper; E-portfolio, WEB-portfolio). The paper format (binder) has been chosen for its ease of application. Make sure your portfolio is well organised and easy to read.

THE CONCEPT OF TUTORING

At the start of each placement, you will be under the direct supervision of a university hospital teacher called a tutor, appointed by the head of department, for the duration of the placement.

As a tutor, you will be required to :

▶ Demonstrate seriousness and professionalism.

▶ Embracing the concept of tutoring by establishing a relationship conducive to exchange

▶ fuctuous with your tutor.

▶ Be active, and show the will to be at the centre of your vocation.

▶ Regularly ensure that the pace of learning activities is maintained: at the

▶ At least one validated RSCA per month is strongly encouraged.

▶ Diversify the themes of learning activities.

Voh-e hJteur, pouna, at your request:

▶ You coach and supervise voh-e acquisition of skills and various learning activities

▶ To guide you in :

Conection/discussion of clinical cases presented at staff meetings.

Helping you to acquire skills during your placement by visiting patients' beds, supervising procedures and...

You will have monthly meetings with your supervisor during your placement.

· At the first interview, you will introduce yourself to your tutor. You bring your portfolio so that the tutor can assess your progress. You express your felt needs and expectations in relation to the placement. Together, you discuss any difficulties or gaps in relation to your stage of progress on the course. Together, you set out the skills you will need to acquire and the objectives you hope to achieve during the placement.

· Subsequent interviews will provide an opportunity to discuss or clarify clinical case studies of hospital patients (learning clinical reasoning, clarifying grey areas: key elements of the diagnosis, etc.). During each interview, you are also invited to present your new learning activities, in particular the RSCA and the logbook. The tutor validates (or not) the learning activity presented. If the work is not validated, you will have to do further research and rectify your learning activity and have it revalidated by your tutor at the next interview.

-At the end of the placement, you discuss with your tutor whether or not you have achieved the objectives you set yourself at the beginning of the placement, what difficulties you have encountered and what challenges you have overcome.

EVALUATION

Portfolio assessment

At the end of each placement, the tutor will write a reasoned opinion in the portfolio. This opinion will take into account various parameters:

-Keeping appointments and the quality of tutor-tutor exchanges.

-Support for the tutoring system.

-Quality o f analysis of complex clinical situations, with a particular emphasis on reflexivity

-All the documents making up the portfolio.

Validation of the course

At the end of the placement, the head of department, in consultation with the tutor, is required to issue a placement validation certificate. This validation includes assessment of the portfolio and covers:

-Your practical and theoretical learning.

-Your relations with medical and paramedical staff and peers.

-Your support for the p01tfolio educational system.

-Voh-e progress during the course.

"Your portfolio should be an authentic reflection of your career and your aspirations. It should tell your story in a unique and engaging way. To help you structure your thoughts, we have provided a sample outline below. **Don't hesitate to adapt it** to suit your specific needs and fütufs projects. This plan is only a suggestion, and we encourage you to give free rein to your creativity."

1. Identification sheet

It is like an identity card that can be consulted by the placement tutor or referee. It includes a photograph, your contact details (telephone, e-mail address, address, etc.) and a "student" mini-curriculum vitae. It also includes the internship course (placements already completed).

-First and last name

-Date and place of birth

-National identity card number

-Address

-Civil status

-Email

-Telephone p01table

Internship programme

Period	Internship

2. Learning activities -

Learning activities can be varied. As active learning and reflection are strongly recommended, we will look in detail at two activities: recounting complex authentic situations, internship diaries, etc.

As mentioned above, each learning activity included in your portfolio must be justified (interest, relevance, etc.) and followed by a reflection.

Authentic Complex Situation Report (ACSR):

You must write at least !stories per month, i.e. 4 stories during the placement period, which you must validate with your tutor. Each story must have a title, and the date and location of the clinical situation must also be specified. It is not a "clinical observation" in the medical sense of the term: it is a reflection on a situation that you have personally experienced in the course of your daily practice. The script has five parts: the narrative, the analysis, the skills required and learning tasks, the summary and finally the references. It combines description and reflection on a complex, authentic situation, giving details of the problems posed, the knowledge required, the skills involved and the changes observed in professional practice.

The five components of an RSCA :

1 The story describing the situation
-The situation: where and when did it happen? -Meeting the patient: biopsychosocial elements who is he? What did he tell me about his history and pathology? What did his clinical examination tell me? -Patient care and outcome: what happened? -My feelings
2) L'analyse (autoévaluation de ma pratique
-Were the decisions I made valid (evidence-based medicine)? The scientific knowledge at my disposal : What scientific data was available? What was the level of evidence Were they up to date ,r.Clinical circumstances : Have they influenced my decisions ,r.The patient (wishes, representations) Have I taken this into account in my approach to care? The doctor's competence: Have I had problems with my professional skills? Have I had problems with my personality? Have I considered my doubts and uncertainties? -What problems have I encountered? I'm asking questions that I think need to be looked at in greater depth.I'm doing a literature search Have I described it correctly? (Books, notes, key words...) Did I laugh at the level of proof?
3) The skills needed in this situation and the associated learning tasks. learning tasks self-training -My acquired skills: what skills have I used? -Skills to be acquired: what skills have I missed out on? -My learning tasks: how can I acquire these skills?
4) La synthèse (le rétroviseur
What did I learn? Is what I have learned applicable to the patient and the situation described? Is what I have learned likely to change my approach? Write them according to the Vancouver recommendations

Internship diary:

This is a collection of memorable situations and/or one-off or specific events that struck you during your placement.

Key situation	Type of difficulty encountered	Documentary reference	Research summary	CAT faced with a situation analogue	Tutor instruction
Case 1					
Case 2					
Case 3					
Case 4					

3. **Skills acquired**

The following table will help you identify the skills you have already acquired and those on which you would like to focus more. Don't hesitate to discuss your progress and ask for regular feedback to make sure you're achieving your training objectives.

Category	Skills	Level Acquisition (1-S)	Comment	Objectives of progress
General skills	Mastery of scientific fundamentals			
	Application of the methods scientists			
	Professional communication			
	Working in a team multidisciplinary			
	Compliance with ethical and deontolo!!:i□ues principles			
Skills specific to HGE	Medical history and physical examination			
	- Paraclinical evaluation: Interpretation of biological tests Imaging Endoscopy			
	- Diagnosis: Making the diagnosis of digestive emergencies			
	- Therapeutics: Prescribing and managing treatments for common pathologics in HGE			
	- Prevention: Identification risk factors, health promotion, screening			
	- Technical procedures: Mastery of specific technical procedures Ascites puncture Nasogastric tube			

4. Library and personal research

This section contains all the documents you have been looking for to help you resolve the various difficult issues you have had to face during your placement: articles, updates, recommendations from learned societies, etc.

5. Internship report

In this section you will describe :

- Reasons for choosing the internship te1rnin ;
- The training objectives of this course ;
- The positive and negative aspects of the course;
- Objectives achieved and those not achieved;
- The new training objectives at the end of this course.

6. FREE SPACE

This is a space for you to express yourself freely in relation to your overall self-assessment and your experience of the placement, the difficulties you encountered, any experiences or events that stood out, and any criticisms and suggestions for improving your own learning experience as part of the team.

SUMMARY

Introduction: *Recent reforms to the medical education system in Tunisia have emphasised the acquisition of clinical skills and the development of a learner-centred approach. In this context, the portfolio appears to be a relevant pedagogical tool to support interns in their training.*

Objective: To *draw up a portfolio guide for interns at the Faculty of Medicine in Sousse assigned to the hepato-gastroenterology (HGE) department in order to implement it in the clinical environment.*

Methods: *A literature review was carried out to identify best practice in portfolios in the medical field. In addition, an in-depth analysis of the current state of training for interns in the HGE department was used to identify the specific needs of this group.*

Results: *The study resulted in the creation of a portfolio guide for interns assigned to the HGE department. This guide clearly defines the objectives of the portfolio, detailing its content and application methods. It proposes a structure comprising an identification form, learning activities such as accounts of complex authentic situations and the internship diary, as well as a space dedicated to personal reflection. Rigorous assessment criteria have also been devised to evaluate interns' clinical and interpersonal skills, as well as their ability to self-evaluate.*

Conclusion: *This work has made it possible to draw up a personalised portfolio guide for interns assigned to the HGE department, thus meeting a specific need in medical training. A pilot phase will enable the guide to be adjusted in the light of feedback from interns and tutors.*

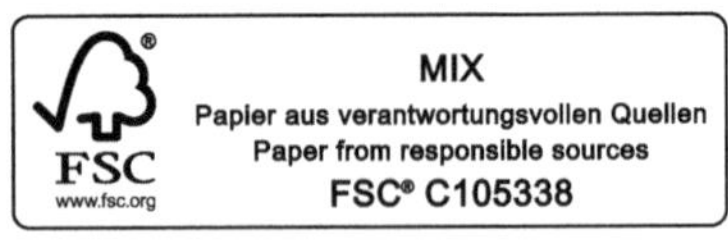

Printed by Books on Demand GmbH, Norderstedt / Germany